NEW
MEDICATIONS

The Debate
Over Approval
and Access

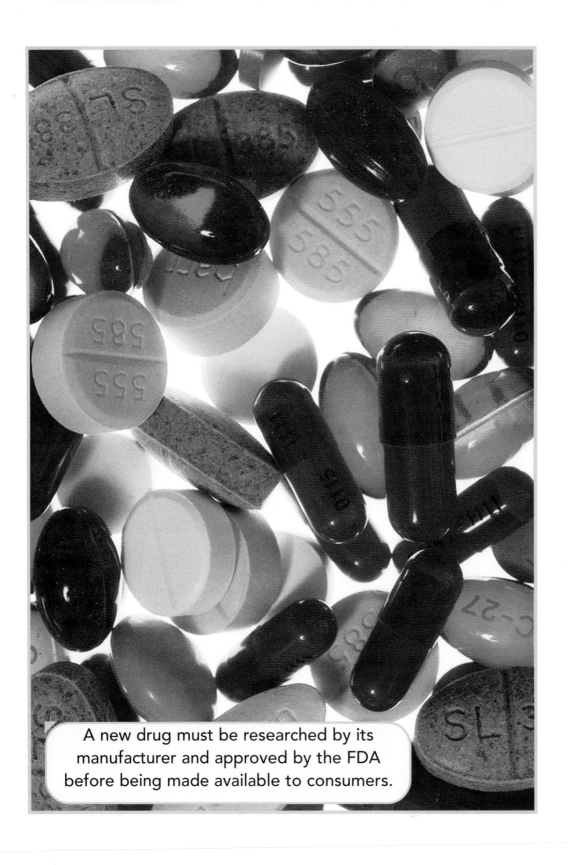

A new drug must be researched by its manufacturer and approved by the FDA before being made available to consumers.

NEW MEDICATIONS

The Debate Over Approval and Access

Debbie Stanley

THE ROSEN PUBLISHING GROUP, INC.

Published in 2000 by The Rosen Publishing Group, Inc.
29 East 21st Street, New York, NY 10010

First Edition

Library of Congress Cataloging-in-Publication Data

Stanley, Debbie.
   New Medications : the debate over approval and access / Debbie Stanley.
     p. cm. — (Focus on science and society)
   Includes bibliographical references and index.
   Summary: Discusses the ethical issues surrounding the Food and Drug Administration's regulation of the testing, marketing, and sale of drugs in the United States.
   ISBN 0-8239-3212-5
   1. Drugs—Research—Juvenile literature. 2. Drugs—Law and legislation—United States—Juvenile literature. 3. United States—Food and Drug Administration—Juvenile literature. 4. Health services accessibility—United States—Juvenile literature. [1. Drugs—Research. 2. Drugs—Law and legislation. 3. United States—Food and Drug Administration. 4. Health services accessibility.]
   I. Title. II. Series.
   RS122 .S72 2000
   615'.19—dc21
                                        00-020571

Manufactured in the United States of America

CONTENTS

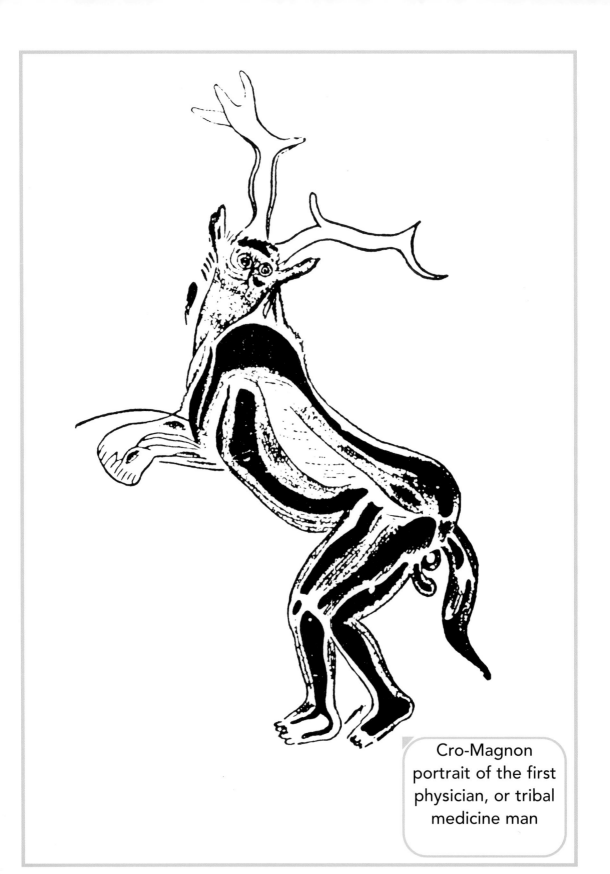

Cro-Magnon portrait of the first physician, or tribal medicine man

INTRODUCTION
MEDICINE THROUGHOUT HISTORY

People have been medicating themselves since the beginning of time. Researchers studying remains found by archaeologists have learned that prehistoric peoples had varying degrees of expertise in the use of herbs and other plants to ease their aches, pains, and physical or mental irritations. Many of today's modern medicines are derived from these ancient treatments.

For thousands of years in Eastern cultures, and as far back as 400 BC in Western civilization, there were people who were able to heal others by using techniques and substances that had been found to improve or cure various conditions. Hippocrates (pronounced Hip-AH-crah-tees), a Greek physician who is considered the father of Western medicine, lived from 460 to 377 BC and is credited with separating religion, superstition, and philosophy from the practice of medicine, focusing instead on the rational and scientific aspects of the operation of the human body.

NEW MEDICATIONS

Thomas Sydenham, a physician of the seventeenth century, is credited with reintroducing the Hippocratic approach to the practice of medicine; for this reason, Sydenham is also known as the "English Hippocrates."

Hippocrates and Sydenham both made use of many different techniques and methods to help their patients, but among the most important were medications. In fact, aspirin, the most basic of modern drugs, was prescribed by Hippocrates in its original form, a potion derived from the bark and leaves of the willow tree. More drugs were invented, discovered, or refined over the centuries, and in many cases they led to the healing or easing of symptoms. Today there are many different types of "doctoring" being practiced in the world. Besides the mainstream medical training that leads to a person becoming an M.D. or specialist, there are also programs in fields such as homeopathy, herbal

Timeline

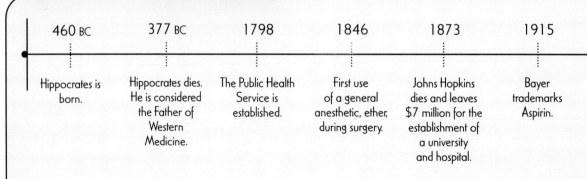

460 BC	377 BC	1798	1846	1873	1915
Hippocrates is born.	Hippocrates dies. He is considered the Father of Western Medicine.	The Public Health Service is established.	First use of a general anesthetic, ether, during surgery.	Johns Hopkins dies and leaves $7 million for the establishment of a university and hospital.	Bayer trademarks Aspirin.

medicine, Asian arts (which include techniques such as acupuncture), and even practices with religious or superstitious connotations. All of these systems have proponents and patients who use them to heal illness and injury. What they all have in common is the use of substances intended to aid the healing process— substances that, loosely defined, could be considered medicines.

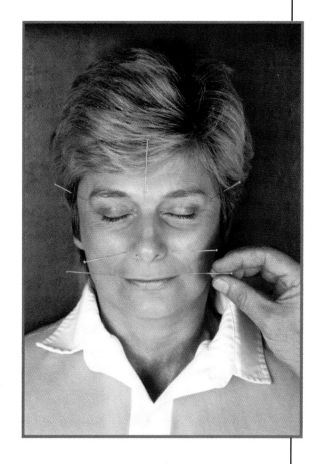

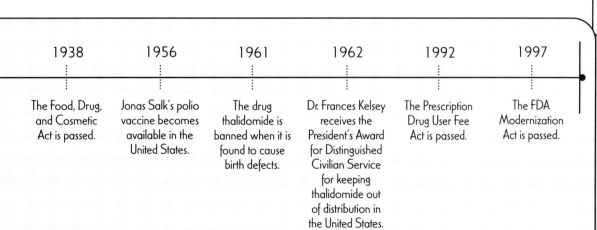

1938	1956	1961	1962	1992	1997
The Food, Drug, and Cosmetic Act is passed.	Jonas Salk's polio vaccine becomes available in the United States.	The drug thalidomide is banned when it is found to cause birth defects.	Dr. Frances Kelsey receives the President's Award for Distinguished Civilian Service for keeping thalidomide out of distribution in the United States.	The Prescription Drug User Fee Act is passed.	The FDA Modernization Act is passed.

Abuse of Medicine

Early on, some people realized that they could make a lot of money by selling "medicines" to desperate people, promising to heal them with products that in fact did nothing to change their conditions or, in some cases, even made them worse. The products were usually sold by traveling salesmen or self-proclaimed "doctors" who described their potions as exotic concoctions from faraway places, with secret recipes or even magical properties. Sharp consumers who saw through the scams dubbed these fake medicines "snake oil" and referred to their providers as "snake oil salesmen." By the eighteenth century, it had become clear that the practice of medicine, unregulated as it was, could be dangerous to the public. The U.S. Department of Health and Human Services responded by establishing the Public Health Service in 1798. The Public Health Service, in turn, oversees the Food and Drug Administration (FDA), which was created to administer the Food, Drug, and Cosmetic Act of 1938. The FDA is charged with ensuring that all drugs, whether prescription or over-the-counter, are safe and effective for Americans to use. Since the FDA began regulating the testing, marketing, and sale of drugs in the United States, many questions and ethical issues have arisen. The FDA's approval process and Americans' access to new drugs are much debated and contested topics.

PIONEERS: HIPPOCRATES

Hippocrates was a Greek physician who lived from around 460 BC to 377 BC. The Hippocratic Oath, the promise every physician makes before beginning to treat patients, is named after Hippocrates. Hippocrates is considered the father of Western medicine because he changed the way disease was seen by doctors and patients alike. Before his time, disease was believed to be the result of having angered the gods or of failing to abide by a variety of superstitions; treatment included more superstitious behavior, and even sacrifices. Hippocrates instead demonstrated that disease was most often the result of an unhealthy environment. Circumstances that had previously never been considered, such as the quality of a town's drinking water or the presence of rats, were linked to illness through impartial scientific investigation.

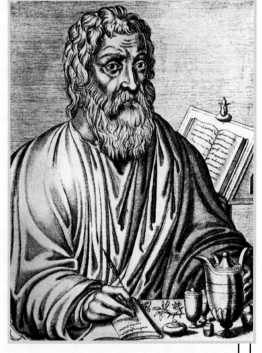

The prevailing theory that came from the "Hippocratic" method of treating patients was that of the "four humors." This theory, which has nothing to do with the concept of humor or comedy as we know it today, asserted that illness occurred when there was an imbalance in the body caused by an excess of one of the four humors. These "humors," or bodily substances, were yellow bile, black bile, phlegm, and blood. Each was associated with one of the four seasons and with one of the four elements: Yellow bile goes with summer and fire; black bile goes with autumn and earth; phlegm goes with winter and water; and blood goes with spring and air. The treatments derived from this theory called for the physician to first determine which element was dominating and then try to increase its opposite. For example, a Hippocratic doctor would prescribe wine for an excess of phlegm (for example, a cold) and cold baths for an excess of yellow bile (for example, a fever). Much of this system still makes at least some sense in modern times.

Another health concern pioneered by Hippocrates was that of preventive medicine. Taking what was then a radical stance, Hippocrates insisted that a person's diet, lifestyle, and attitude were important contributors to his or her health—another concept that stands up to the scrutiny of modern medicine.

CASE STUDY: ASPIRIN

Aspirin is often referred to as a "wonder drug," and with good reason: Despite a history of more than 2,400 years of use and hundreds of attempts to imitate it, aspirin is still the simplest way to ease pain, reduce fever and swelling, and prevent heart attack and stroke.

Aspirin (technically acetylsalicylic acid) is derived from the bark of the willow tree. As such, its use can be traced as far back as the ancient Greeks and Native Americans. A German chemist named Felix Hoffman made aspirin truly useful for the general population. Hoffman, who worked for Bayer (one of today's most easily recognized brand names), wanted to find a way to improve sodium salicylate, a sort of "rough draft" of modern-day aspirin used as a pain reliever in the 1800s. He was motivated by the pain he saw his father enduring, both from arthritis and from the stomach problems caused by the sodium salicylate he took to relieve his arthritis symptoms. Hoffman found success around the turn of the century, but reports differ as to how he did it: Some say he himself synthesized acetylsalicylic acid, which was trademarked by Bayer as the brand name Aspirin in 1915, while others say he rediscovered the work of French chemist Charles Frederic Gerhardt, who is believed to have created the same compound approximately fifty years earlier but failed to see the value in marketing it.

Today, aspirin, which lost its capital A when Bayer had to give up its trademark as part of Germany's World War II war reparations, is used to treat pain, fever, and swelling due to injuries, arthritis, and other inflammatory diseases. Its blood-thinning properties are believed to help prevent heart attacks, reduce damage during a heart attack, and lower the risk of stroke, colon cancer, and preeclampsia (a life-threatening complication of pregnancy). Aspirin does have side effects, however; besides the stomach-irritation problem that still plagues it, aspirin has also been linked with an increased risk of Reye's syndrome in children, and it must never be given to people with blood disorders such as hemophilia or those who take other blood-thinning drugs.

Author's Note

In all cases throughout this book, the medications being discussed are either drugs that are legal for over-the-counter or prescription use, or drugs that are not yet approved for use but, if approved, will be allowed for medicinal use. The use of the term "drugs" in this book never refers to or includes illegal drugs such as marijuana, cocaine, heroin, or other recreational drugs, or illegal uses of legal drugs, such as the abuse of tranquilizers as date rape drugs.

CHAPTER 1

HOW NEW DRUGS ARE DEVELOPED

Many people decide during childhood that they want to be doctors in order to find a cure for cancer, AIDS, or other life-threatening or incurable diseases. Those who follow through on this dream often become research scientists working toward the discovery of new drugs or different uses for existing ones. Many of those research scientists work for pharmaceutical companies (the companies that develop drugs), working on new formulas, modifying old ones, and conducting research to present to the FDA so that the new medications can be approved for distribution in the United States.

Development, Research, and Testing

There are dozens of pharmaceutical companies in the United States, all engaged in the research and development of new medicines and the improvement of old ones. These companies are generally publicly held, meaning that anyone can buy stock in them, and they are in business to make a profit. In other words, they are not nonprofit or charitable organizations. This does not necessarily mean, however, that making money is their primary goal. It is up to consumers—the people who use their products—to decide whether a pharmaceutical company (or any service-oriented company) operates from a desire to help humankind or simply from greed.

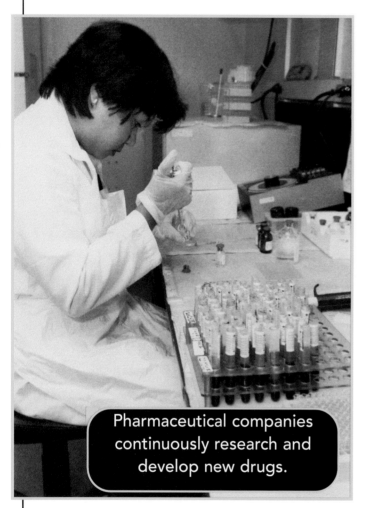

Pharmaceutical companies continuously research and develop new drugs.

It is important to note that, although the FDA oversees the drugs made available to Americans, it does not itself do the research and development of these drugs. Instead, it reviews the research completed by the

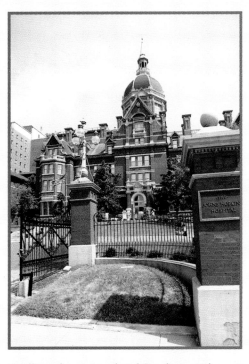

PIONEERS: JOHNS HOPKINS

Johns Hopkins was not a doctor, but he made a significant impact on the future of medicine in the United States. Hopkins, born in 1795, was a financier who made his fortune in banking and investing. When he died in 1873, he left $7 million to build a university and a hospital. Located in Baltimore, Maryland, Johns Hopkins University was founded in 1876 and its School of Medicine opened in 1893; Johns Hopkins Hospital, a groundbreaking medical facility and training ground for Johns Hopkins University's students, opened in 1889.

Johns Hopkins Medicine, the collective name for the university, hospital, and medical school, is credited with a great number of inventions, discoveries, improvements, modifications, and new standards of practice that have improved medical care in the last 100 years. Among its drug-related achievements are the isolation of epinephrine (1897); the discovery of the blood-thinner heparin (1916-18); development of the antiseptic mercurochrome (1919); discovery of vitamin D (1922); development of oral rehydration therapy (1960s); identification of drug receptors in the brain, important information for the treatment of drug addiction, and the development of nonaddictive painkillers (1973, 1987); and discovery of the value of vitamin A in combating blindness (1983-86).

> Johns Hopkins Medicine remains on the cutting edge of medical technology, continuing to research new ways to improve quality of life for sick people, prevent illness in those who are well, and teach medical professionals to provide excellent care for their patients—all thanks to a gift from a philanthropic businessperson.

manufacturers; after a drug is approved, the FDA oversees follow-up research and requires certain post-approval reviews. The clinical testing, or testing on humans, that must be performed in order for a drug to gain FDA approval is an area of controversy. Many people who are unable to afford treatment for their health problems actively seek out clinical trials in which to participate in order to receive some medication for at least a short while. This practice, in which people with no other options use clinical trials as their sole means of health care, is considered by some to be a glaring example of everything that is wrong with the U.S. health care system. Others worry that if tests are populated primarily with "drug trial nomads," the results may not be representative of the average American.

While it may not be perfect, the practice of using volunteers for testing is certainly an improvement over methods of the past, in which prisoners and people held in insane asylums were reportedly used in experiments against their will or without their knowledge of what was being done to them. Such barbaric practices were also used on prisoners in the death camps of the Holocaust. Society did, in many cases, benefit from these inhumane experiments, and some people today believe that death-row prisoners should be required to repay their debt to society by being used as human test subjects before they are executed.

FDA Approval

Once a new drug has been researched and its manufacturer is ready to make it available for sale, the manufacturer must submit an application for approval to the FDA. The FDA reviews medications that are consistent with traditional Western medicine. Another government agency, the National Center for Complementary and Alternative Medicine, researches and investigates alternative modes of treatment such as holistic medicine, homeopathy, nutritional therapy, and chiropractic medicine.

Another hot topic is the future of homeopathic remedies, which are currently not required to undergo FDA approval. Patients and practitioners of homeopathic medicine are divided over whether or not their remedies should fall under the FDA's authority. Some believe the standardization and rigorous testing required

CASE STUDY: ETHER

It's hard to believe, but up until the first half of the 1800s, people endured surgery while awake and with little or no relief from the pain. The discovery that a liquid called ether (pronounced EE-ther) could be used to ren-

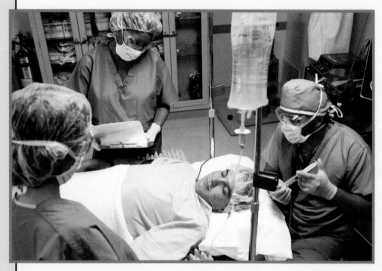

der patients unconscious and spare them the experience of pain during surgery has been described as medicine's greatest gift to humankind.

Credit for the first documented use of ether in surgery goes to William T. G. Morton, a Boston dentist, who demonstrated its effectiveness in a procedure performed on October 16, 1846, in front of a group of astonished physicians and medical students. Morton administered the ether by having the patient inhale its vapors from a saturated sponge; when the patient no longer responded and seemed unaware of his surroundings, noted surgeon John Collins Warren removed a tumor from the patient's jaw. Another surgeon, Henry J. Bigelow, documented the procedure in an article published in the *Boston Medical and Surgical Journal* and reported that the patient indicated that he had felt some pain, but that the medication had blunted it. In another surgery performed the next day, a second patient reported no pain and no awareness of her surroundings during the procedure.

Bigelow attributed the first patient's moderate pain to "some defect in the process of inhalation" during the first operation.

Great strides have been made in the field of anesthesiology since that first procedure, but to the people of the 1800s, who lived in fear of ever needing an operation, the invention was a miracle. The London *People's Journal* declared the importance of "this noble discovery of the power to still the sense of pain, and veil the eye and memory from all the horrors of an operation."

would protect patients; others fear that such regulation would increase prices of remedies that are generally quite inexpensive and would restrict many remedies to availability only by prescription, effectively eliminating the consumer's ability to self-medicate.

CHAPTER 2

ACCESS ISSUE: FDA APPROVAL

In order for a drug to be legally sold in the United States, it must be approved by the Food and Drug Administration (FDA). On its Web site, the FDA describes its job as "to see that the food we eat is safe and wholesome, the cosmetics we use won't hurt us, the medicines and medical devices we use are safe and effective, and that radiation-emitting products such as microwave ovens won't do us harm." Pharmaceutical companies must

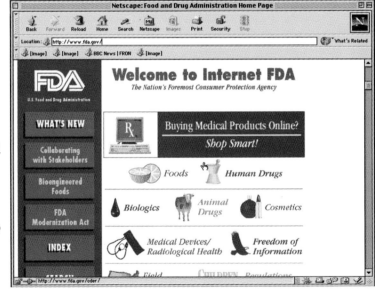

submit an application for each new drug they create, along with research findings that, they hope, will satisfy the FDA's requirements for safety and effectiveness. The FDA reports that its "approximately 9,000 employees monitor the manufacture, import, transport, storage and sale of about $1 trillion worth of products each year."

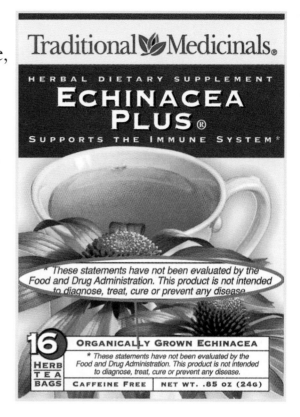

FDA Requirements

While the FDA's primary responsibility is to ensure that the drugs and other products under its jurisdiction are safe and effective for consumers, it emphasizes that "safe" does not mean completely risk-free. The amount of risk, in the form of negative side effects, that is allowed in a drug depends on the severity of the condition it is treating and the amount of benefit the drug is expected to deliver. The FDA addresses the question of benefit versus risk on its Web site, stating, "Benefit to risk evaluation at the time of approval is largely qualitative and contextual. That is, depending on the disease

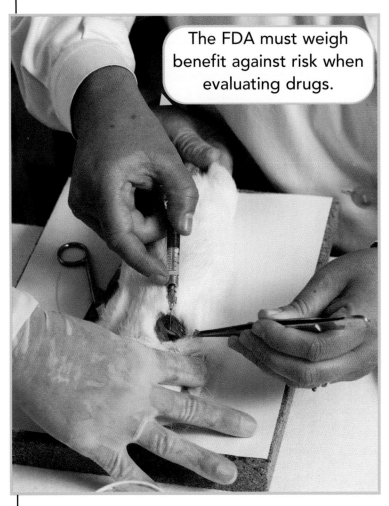

The FDA must weigh benefit against risk when evaluating drugs.

being treated, different degrees of risk are tolerated and the degree of benefit is not necessarily uniform in all cases. For example, in treating cancer a great deal of risk is tolerated for, at times, a small incremental benefit. Conversely, for a drug approved to treat simple headache, the benefit is real but the risk tolerance is very low."

The first step in developing a new drug, after it is invented or discovered, is to conduct early research and "preclinical" testing, meaning testing that is not performed on humans. The Pharmaceutical Research and Manufacturers of America (PhRMA), a group representing approximately

100 U.S. pharmaceutical companies, reports that this stage of development takes an average of six to seven years. This research and testing is often performed on animals, a fact that provokes constant protest and sometimes even violence from animal rights activists.

After preclinical testing is completed, the first submission is made to the FDA. The pharmaceutical company files an Investigational New Drug Application, or IND, with the FDA in order to receive approval to begin testing the drug in humans. The IND includes an explanation of what the drug is intended to do, how it is believed to work, how it is manufactured, and the methods

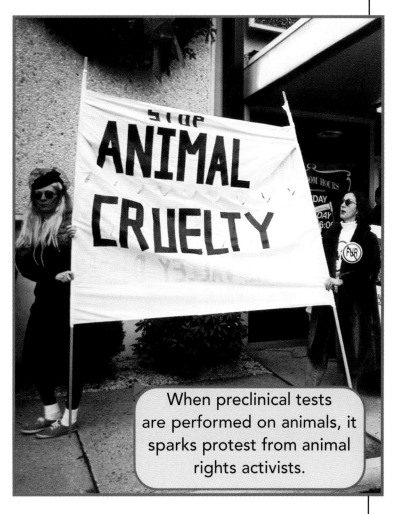

When preclinical tests are performed on animals, it sparks protest from animal rights activists.

and results of all research done so far. If the FDA does not deny the IND application within thirty days, it is automatically approved and human trials may begin.

A new drug must go through at least three phases of clinical trials, in which volunteers take the drug and are monitored so researchers can determine the safe dosage range, any side effects, and whether or not the drug does what it is supposed to do. In the first phase, a small group of normal, healthy people (usually fewer than 100 participants) are given the drug and are monitored to determine its effects on them. In the second phase, a larger group of volunteers (from 100 to 300 people) who have the condition the drug was developed to treat take the drug. In the third phase, a much larger group (from 1,000 to 3,000 patients) receives the drug. The PhRMA reports that the clinical testing stage takes another six to seven years, although in the case of drugs in high demand, manufacturers often work to streamline the process and eliminate delays. This research must be analyzed and drawn together in a New Drug Application (NDA), which is submitted to the FDA, and the countdown to public access begins.

Timeline to Approval

It used to take much longer than it now does for a drug to work its way through the FDA approval process. The Prescription Drug User Fee Act of 1992 (PDUFA) led to a

PIONEERS: FRANCES KELSEY

Americans have Frances Kelsey to thank for protecting them from a drug with horrendous side effects.

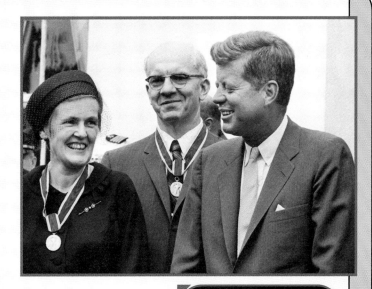

Kelsey was a brand-new member of the Food and Drug Administration staff when thalidomide's application for approval came under the scrutiny of the FDA. The drug was to be marketed as a treatment for the nausea, commonly known as morning sickness, that leaves many pregnant women miserable and un-

Frances Kelsey saved people from thalidomide's side effects.

able to eat. The drug was already widely used in Europe and was doing what it promised to do. Thinking the application would be a simple one to review and would give her an easy introduction to her new job, Kelsey's superiors at the FDA gave her the thalidomide application to process.

At that time, standard practice was to approve a drug after sixty days unless the FDA found a compelling reason to delay it. Thalidomide's distributors were expecting to be able to sell the drug after two months and were eager to do so. Since it had proven effective in other countries, they anticipated that there would be many grateful customers among pregnant American women.

Imagine the uproar when Kelsey, a new agent, refused to approve the application. She cited concerns over inadequate testing of the drug, despite the distributor's insistence that it had tested thalidomide and found it safe in lab animals. However, they had not tested it on pregnant animals, and to Kelsey's mind, this meant it should not be given to pregnant women without further study. Although her concern was for the public good, many people resented her interference. Public outrage over Kelsey's "bureaucratic nitpicking," as one newspaper called it, grew steadily stronger.

Nonetheless, Kelsey weathered the storm and resisted approving thalidomide, holding out until the tragic consequences of its use in other countries became known and it was removed from distribution in 1961. At that point, her caution was finally found to be justified and Kelsey quickly went from being ostracized as a heartless troublemaker to being hailed as a hero. Kelsey was awarded the United States President's Award for Distinguished Civilian Service in 1962.

In the same year that President John F. Kennedy presented Kelsey with the President's Award, the thalidomide disaster prompted Congress to enact legislation that set strict rules for the testing and approval of drugs to be marketed in the United States. The Drug Amendments Act of 1962 gave the FDA more power, and the FDA in turn began requiring drug manufacturers to prove that their products have no effect on fetal development. The FDA has since maintained its position as overseer of the drugs approved for distribution to Americans.

shorter approval process by providing additional funding to the FDA, paid in the form of user fees by pharmaceutical companies. The FDA reports that the additional funds led to managerial reforms and the addition of 696 employees. However, critics say that these improvements are still not enough. The FDA is legally required to complete its review of an NDA within six months, but it has traditionally failed to meet this goal. In 1997, for example, the FDA reported that its average review period was fifteen months, which cut in half the thirty-month average of the pre-PDUFA years. Consumers are left to weigh the question of whether the FDA should be allowed to work at its own pace in the interest of completing a thorough review, or whether it should be forced to comply with the six-month rule and possibly produce work of lesser quality. It is important to note that a typical NDA is not just a report in a little plastic folder: The PhRMA estimates that an average NDA is 100,000 pages long.

The FDA states that it is committed to increasing patient access to experimental drugs and accelerating the review process for important new medications. These improvements were among the purposes of the FDA Modernization Act of 1997. Whether this goal has been accomplished is, again, left to consumers and industry experts to decide. However, there have been a number of cases in which the FDA has granted conditional early approval, allowing patients to receive new drugs before all research on them has been completed.

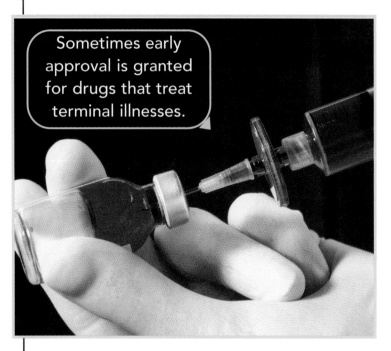

Sometimes early approval is granted for drugs that treat terminal illnesses.

This policy change was implemented largely in response to the emergence of AIDS. John Henkel, writing in the FDA's *FDA Consumer Magazine*, reports, "Under the agency's accelerated approval regulations, a drug can be marketed without studies that show direct effects on clinical disease progression or death. Instead, the FDA relies on 'surrogate markers,' such as viral load, which are laboratory measurements intended to reliably predict a drug's ultimate clinical benefit." In order to qualify for accelerated approval, a drug must meet three criteria: the "surrogate marker" must be considered a reliable predictor of actual benefit; the manufacturer must agree to complete postmarketing studies that will generate data proving the drug's effectiveness; and the manufacturer must prove the drug's benefit within a reasonable time after the early access begins.

What Happens After Approval?

The FDA requires certain post-approval reviews and research, some of which is especially extensive, depending on the drug; even after they have been approved, many drugs remain controversial and are regarded with suspicion. An example is thalidomide, a drug that was found to cause

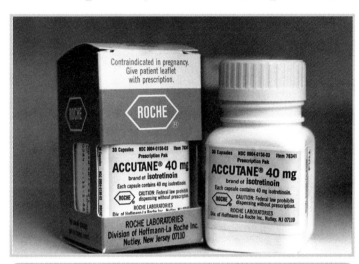

The acne drug Accutane, like thalidomide, can cause birth defects when used improperly.

birth defects and has been refused FDA approval since the 1960s. After almost forty years of exile, thalidomide was recently approved for extremely limited use. While the drug has been extensively studied and holds promise as a treatment for a handful of conditions, it is still capable of causing devastating birth defects. As often happens with controversial, unapproved drugs, a black market for thalidomide had sprung up, and birth defects attributable to thalidomide use were occurring once again.

Randolph Warren, an adult survivor of thalidomide and

CASE STUDY: THALIDOMIDE

This drug is an extreme example of what can happen when a medication is not thoroughly tested before it is released to the public. In fact, thalidomide is considered the main reason that there are now such strict regulations.

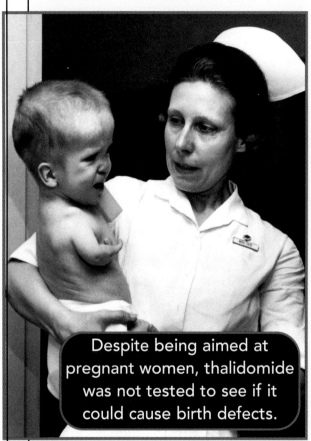

Despite being aimed at pregnant women, thalidomide was not tested to see if it could cause birth defects.

Thalidomide was introduced in 1957 as a sedative, and soon became popular for its ability to alleviate the nausea and vomiting that often occur in pregnant women. Thalidomide's manufacturer, Chemie Grunenthal of Germany, claimed that its safety had been proven through testing on lab animals. The company's testing, however, had been inadequate: Despite the fact that it was marketing the drug specifically for pregnant women, no tests had been performed on pregnant animals. The drug was sold in over forty countries both by prescription and over the counter. As a result, over 10,000 babies were born with a severe birth defect called phocomelia, which affects the limbs. The condition caused some children to be born with flippers extending from their shoulders instead of arms; others had no legs, just toes protruding from their hips; others were born with no limbs at all—just a head and torso. Many were also afflicted with heart problems or abnormalities of other internal organs.

Thalidomide had a devastating impact in European countries, but Americans were protected from it by the FDA and its agent Dr. Frances Kelsey. Kelsey blocked approval of the drug and prevented its distribution here. When the connection between the drug and the seeming epidemic of birth defects was finally made in 1961, thalidomide was withdrawn from worldwide distribution.

Despite its horrific early history, thalidomide may still prove beneficial for some conditions. It is currently approved for treatment of a few rare conditions, such as leprosy, and is being studied for use against macular degeneration (an eye disease); cancers of the brain, breast, and prostate; and Kaposi's sarcoma (a cancer common among AIDS patients). Those patients who are treated with thalidomide are also educated in the strongest possible language to avoid having children while taking the drug. While it may help them fight certain diseases, it is nonetheless still capable of causing debilitating birth defects. Therefore, both male and female patients are warned to use not one but two reliable forms of birth control for many weeks before they begin using thalidomide and until many weeks after they stop taking it.

CEO of the Thalidomide Victims Association of Canada (TVAC), has stated that the reemergence of thalidomide put the TVAC in an awkward position. Since the drug was already reaching consumers, but without accompanying warnings, the TVAC did the unthinkable: It agreed to support efforts to win FDA approval of the drug because such approval would take thalidomide's distribution out of the black market and would necessitate extensive legitimate research. Since legal sale of the drug would require unmistakable warnings to avoid pregnancy, FDA approval would actually help to prevent more thalidomide babies. However, the TVAC continues to campaign for research into alternatives to thalidomide. "The return of thalidomide must remain a temporary reality, with the goal of replacing it being the priority," Warren wrote in a position paper entitled "Living in a World with Thalidomide: A New Reality."

Getting Drugs Before the FDA Does

As happened with thalidomide, many drugs reach consumers through illegal means—for example, black market sales made over the Internet. Unapproved uses of approved drugs—called "off-label prescribing"—are also common and not illegal. In this way, doctors are able to give their patients access to drugs that were originally approved for one use but that might have promise in treating other conditions. These gaps in the FDA's influence leave the door open for exploitation and abuse.

Some people believe that the FDA is not needed. Others don't want to wait for a drug to be approved if it might cure their disease or save their life. These people become willing customers to others who sell unapproved drugs illegally. This situation is dangerous enough to begin with, but it is also a golden opportunity for criminals who are interested not in helping people but in taking their money. People who are desperate for a remedy are more vulnerable to believing in "miracle cures" and less inclined to exercise caution and skepticism in their purchases. To put it simply, they will pay any price for a chance to be healed. Despite the FDA's presence in modern health care, the old-time snake oil salesmen are still in operation.

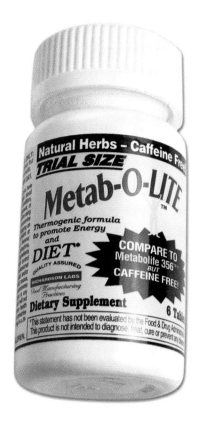

The Internet has increased the reach of these criminals, allowing them to sell their products to people all around the world while hiding behind the anonymity of their Web sites. There is much inaccurate, unfounded, and unresearched information on the Internet, and all legitimate medical groups, including the FDA, strongly recommend that consumers discuss anything they find on the Internet with their doctors before taking action. The FDA maintains an e-mail address for consumers to report suspected fraudulent nonprescription drugs: *otcfraud@cder.fda.gov.*

Yet some people believe that black-market drug providers are actually heroes. Certainly it is plausible that there are people who want to help others and believe that their product is the way to do it but for whatever reason have not taken the legal route to distribution. It is also possible that some of these unapproved products are helpful, but it is much more likely that the number of crooks far surpasses the number of altruistic individuals, and also that the number of dangerous and/or fake unapproved medicines is much greater than the number of such medicines that might actually help or cure a sick person. Still, to desperate people watching a loved one suffer from serious illness or battling it themselves, the hope provided by these black-market sellers is often irresistible.

CHAPTER 3

ACCESS ISSUE: EXPENSE

Medicine costs money. Whether it is paid for by an individual, an employer, an insurance company, or the government, somewhere along the line someone will have to pay for a patient to receive a drug. In the United States, the question of who pays generally comes down to

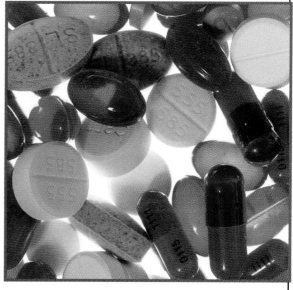

two options: you or your insurance company.

Medicine is also profitable. There are dozens of pharmaceutical manufacturers in the United States, and the amount of money they make is truly astounding. Sales for the third quarter (approximately July through September) of 1999 were reportedly $1.8 billion for Pharmacia & Upjohn, Inc., $5 billion for Bristol-Myers Squibb, $6.7 billion for Johnson & Johnson, and $8.2 billion for Merck & Co. In other words, each of these companies sold over a billion dollars' worth of medicines and medical supplies in just three months.

When You Don't Have Insurance

According to Robert J. Samuelson in the November 8, 1999, issue of *Newsweek*, there are currently 44 million people in the United States who do not have health insurance, either government-provided or through a private insurer. They represent 16 percent of the total population. Of those who are uninsured, 25 percent are children and 40 percent are between the ages of eighteen and thirty-five.

People who do not have insurance sometimes find that they don't need it in the short term. Some people are generally healthy and have good luck in avoiding serious illnesses or injuries. However, they miss out on the important benefit of regular checkups. If they do begin to develop a health problem that is easily detected by a doctor but not always obvious through symptoms, such as high blood pressure, diabetes, or high cholesterol, their diagnosis and treatment will be delayed because they do not see a doctor as often. And when they are diagnosed with such a condition, they quickly discover that the cost of their medications is going to be very high.

For this rea-
son, many people
ignore chronic
health problems
because they
can't afford to
treat them. The
situation becomes
even more des-
perate when the
diagnosis is can-
cer or AIDS—dis-
eases that have a
very poor prognosis

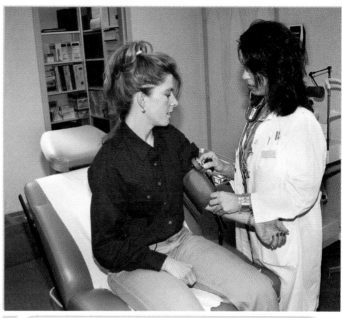

Many people delay in seeing a doctor because they do not have insurance.

without early and aggressive treatment.

Some people react to such news by giving up, believing there is nothing they can do to help themselves.
Others are mobilized by their fear, throwing themselves
into researching alternatives, protesting their lack of
access to expensive treatments, and campaigning to be included in clinical trials of experimental drugs. "In recent
years, the need for test subjects in experimental drug trials has exploded as the industry has brought to market an
ever-increasing number of new products," Gina Kolata and
Kurt Eichenwald reported in the *New York Times*. "In response, drug companies have developed new methods of

PIONEERS: SALK AND SABIN

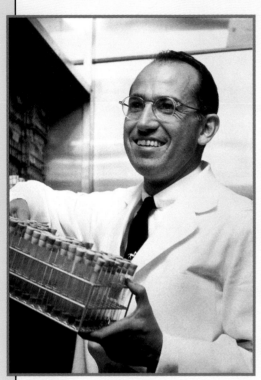

SALK

Drs. Jonas Salk and Albert Sabin share credit for delivering the world from a crippling and sometimes deadly disease: paralytic polio- myelitis, known simply as polio. The word struck fear into the hearts of parents and children living in the 1950s and '60s, when an epidemic of the disease raged with no clear understanding of its cause and no way to prevent or cure it. In 1952, approximately 3,000 people died after contracting polio, and many more were left permanently para- lyzed; an astonishing total of over 57,000 cases of polio were reported. Perhaps the most famous victim of polio was President Franklin Delano Roosevelt, who contracted the disease after already reaching adulthood and spent the rest of his life using a wheelchair or leg braces.

Clearly, there was a desperate need for a way to stop the spread of this horrible disease. Salk set to work and determined that by exposing people to a "killed" version of the polio virus, they could be made immune to infection by the live virus. Salk's polio vaccine was widely used in the United States between 1956 and 1960. During that period, Sabin developed a second polio vaccine, made of live but weakened virus and taken orally instead of by injection. Sabin's vaccine became the preferred method of immunizing against polio because it was easier to administer and because, unlike the Salk vaccine, it did not require follow-up booster shots. Thousands of Americans lined up at their doctor's offices on designated distribution dates—known as Sabin Sundays—to receive a dose of the miracle drug. The vaccine was made available worldwide as well; by 1960, 100 million Europeans had been vaccinated. Sabin refused to patent his vaccine and insisted that it be made available to the world free of charge.

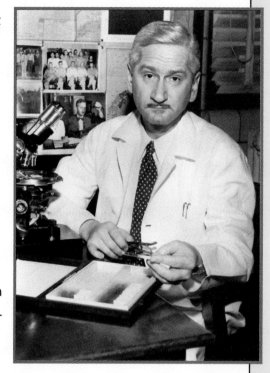

SABIN

Within ten years of the introduction of Salk's and Sabin's vaccines, immunization became a routine part of American life, and the number of polio cases reported in the United States dropped to just a few per year. The need for continued diligence was proven, however, in 1979, when sixteen cases of polio occurred among Amish people in the United States and Canada who had not been vaccinated.

finding participants for the trials by turning to private-practice doctors who recruit from their lists of patients." For some, such programs provide improved quality of life, but their use as treatment is inherently flawed. First, some patients receive the actual drug, while others receive a placebo which contains no medication, and they are not told which they are taking; this is the standard, accepted way of measuring a drug's effects. Second, another purpose of drug trials is to discover any side effects the drug might have; this increases the danger to the test subjects taking the new drug. Finally, drug trials do not continue indefinitely; the drugs are dispensed for a certain amount of time, and when the study ends, so does free access to the drug. "That leaves many patients in a sad position," Kolata and Eichenwald reported. "Having tasted, for a moment, how good life can be when their conditions are controlled, they are plunged back into a life of disabling symptoms."

One last resort exists for people who have no private insurance, are ineligible for government assistance, and have little or no income: indigent drug programs supported by pharmaceutical manufacturers. Most drug companies have such programs, in which they supply medications to doctors to give to patients who have no other way to get them. These programs do not include all drugs, however, and involve sometimes complicated application processes that require a doctor's input. Also, many of the people who need these programs are unaware that they exist.

CASE STUDY: AIDS TREATMENTS

The emergence of HIV infection and its end result, AIDS, brought major changes in the FDA's drug approval process. For the first time, and in response to vocal protests and demonstrations from HIV-positive patients and their supporters, the FDA implemented a system of "accelerated approval"

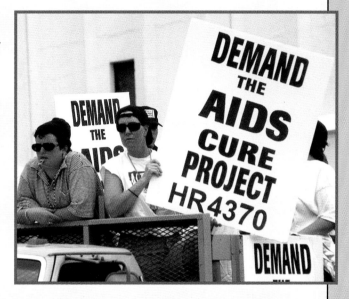

that allows people to try new drugs before they have gone through the complete, formal approval process. The FDA got the message that many people with HIV or AIDS are willing to risk the unknown side effects of a drug that might help them.

The treatment of HIV infection has also brought many changes in the way medicines are administered. The use of "cocktails"—combinations of drugs, each of whose performance is dependent on its interaction with the others—has become the preferred approach, and the drugs used in the cocktails are under constant revision. Researchers continue to search for better, more effective drugs and more precise results from various combinations, with the goal being to prevent the infection from worsening by stopping the virus from replicating within the patient. The desired effect is similar to "remission" in cancer patients, in which the cancer cells stop reproducing and become undetectable in blood tests.

In many cases, the cocktails are doing just that, and in the process giving HIV-infected patients reason to be cautiously optimistic.

Much research is also under way in the search for a vaccine against HIV. Like the polio scare of the 1950s and 1960s, the emergence of AIDS worldwide has marked life in the 1990s. As parents and children shuddered at the mention of polio almost half a century ago, people today live in fear of contracting AIDS. Even though a much better understanding exists of how HIV is spread compared to the relative ignorance of how polio is contracted, people are nonetheless very fearful of being infected with HIV through circumstances beyond their control. While most people know that the primary method of transmission of HIV is unprotected sex, even those who take the recommended precautions still fear infection through a tainted blood transfusion, a rape or other assault resulting in the transfer of bodily fluids, or a doctor's or dentist's use of instruments that have not been properly cleaned and sterilized. Our blood supply is closely monitored, most medical professionals are conscientious in their sterilization techniques, and a single exposure to an HIV-positive person is very unlikely to result in infection in the other person—but these facts do not simply make the worry go away. A vaccine against HIV would be as welcome and as revolutionary as the polio vaccine was almost fifty years ago.

When Insurance Won't Pay

People who have insurance are better off than those who don't, but many are learning at the worst possible time—when they become ill—that having insurance does not mean having unlimited access to treatment and medicines. Many insurance companies will not pay for drugs that are not on their pre-approved list, even if a doctor prescribes them. Most will not cover treatments or medicines considered experimental. These practices limit doctors' treatment choices, forcing them in some cases to prescribe a drug they consider less than ideal for the treatment needed.

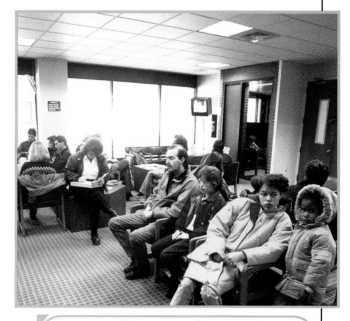

People must often make health choices that have more to do with what they can afford than what they need.

The reality of this situation for many people is that they pay insurance premiums in order to maintain coverage for themselves and their families, yet they also pay exorbitant amounts for medicines that they or their doctors believe they need, but that insurance won't cover. This forces consumers to make choices about their health that have little to do with their needs and everything to do with how much health care they can afford.

Who Are the Bad Guys?

Finger-pointing runs rampant in this debate. Some people say the pharmaceutical manufacturers are to blame for inflating prices; some blame the government for inept management of federally subsidized health care programs; some people believe that health care is a privilege, not a right, and, like any other fee-for-service industry, should be available only to those who can afford it. Opinions tend to be vehement and voiced loudly because everyone feels the impact of the debate in their own lives: Health issues affect—and frighten—everyone personally.

Unfortunately, what is best for one individual may not be best for society as a whole. It often comes down to a question of what is economically sensible versus what is morally right. The result is that people's lives are given a price tag, and often the price is too high to afford.

CHAPTER 4

WHO SHOULD DECIDE?

As you can see from what you've read so far, the debate over access to medicines involves many complex questions and not enough answers. What is your opinion? How do you think drugs should be distributed? Consider what you have read in the preceding chapters, along with other reading or research you've done and discussions you've had with friends, your parents, or with classmates and teachers. Find out how other countries provide medical care, including how drugs are distributed, to its citizens. Then use the following questions to further explore the facts, opinions, and issues involved in this debate. After you've learned even more about the topic of access to drugs in America, you might want to use your knowledge to write a research paper or create a presentation for your science, history, ethics, or government class.

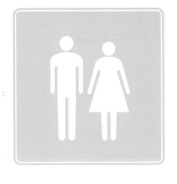

Consumers?

Should consumers—the regular people, like yourself, who will be taking the drug—be given the authority to decide whether or not they should get it? Consider these questions:

- Does the average consumer have the knowledge needed to decide if a drug is safe for himself or herself?

- Should consumers' desire to ease their symptoms or cure their illness be the most important factor in deciding whether they should have access to a drug?

- Should patients be able to override their doctors' decisions?

- Would you consider going to a different country to get a drug that is not available or is much more expensive here?

- Should all medications be available to anyone who wants them, as long as they can afford to pay for them?

- How do you feel about homeopathic remedies, which are available without a prescription and allow consumers to medicate themselves?

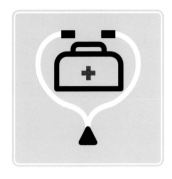

Doctors?

As part of their training, doctors learn how to dispense the drugs that the FDA has made available in this country. But are they qualified to decide whether or not a new drug should be used? Consider these questions:

- Do you think your doctor would have extra time to devote to studying new drugs?

- Do you think doctors would want this responsibility?

- Would each doctor manage his or her own research, or would the work be divided up among all doctors and the results shared?

- What if the doctors chose to concentrate on certain diseases but had little interest in others (for example, rare diseases uncommon in this country)?

- Would the doctors be paid by the drug manufacturers to promote their products? Would this be OK or wrong?

49

- Do you trust your doctor's judgment in what drugs he or she prescribes, and if the FDA did not exist, would you trust him or her to decide which drugs you can and cannot have?

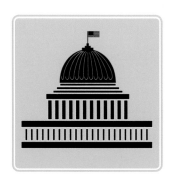

The Government?

Should the United States government have the authority, as it currently does through its Food and Drug Administration, to decide which drugs will be made available to Americans? Consider these questions:

- What effect has the FDA had on Americans' access to drugs?

- Some say the FDA has made legal drug use in this country safer, while others say it has forced people to suffer without a particular drug that might have helped them. What effort has been made to balance these conflicting points?

- What has happened in countries where there is no government regulation of medications? Have there been any problems or negative consequences for patients? Are certain conditions less common or more likely to be cured in countries without government controls?

■ Do you trust the FDA's decisions regarding which drugs you can and cannot have? Do you trust its determination of the amount of risk that is acceptable in a given drug?

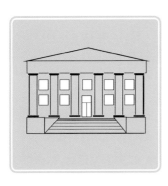

Insurance Companies?

Should insurance companies, the ones who often pay for the drugs their subscribers use, have the authority to decide which drugs their subscribers have access to? Consider these questions:

■ What is the insurance company's goal? In other words, why is it in business?

■ Does the insurance company have enough knowledge of medical issues to make this decision?

■ Some insurance companies have lists of drugs their subscribers are allowed to use and lists of drugs that they will not pay for. Is this right? Which companies do this?

- If your insurance company currently restricts the drugs available to you, do you trust its decisions? If the FDA no longer existed, would you trust your insurance company to decide which drugs you can and cannot have?

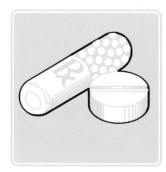

Drug Manufacturers?

Should the companies that make drugs be the ones to decide if their products are safe and who should have access to them? Consider these questions:

- How conscientious are drug companies in performing safety tests? How can you find out if their products have been tested and proven safe?

- How do you feel about the practice of volunteering for clinical trials in order to obtain new, unapproved drugs?

- Are there any conflicts of interest present that might cause the company to downplay or ignore risks?

- Would you trust drug manufacturers to decide which drugs are made available to you?

The issue of access to medications in the United States is steeped in controversy. Many of the debates, arguments, and facts related to this issue have been presented here, but even more could be written. In particular, much can be learned from other countries' approaches to health care—especially countries, such as Canada and Great Britain, in which insurance is provided by the government and costs to the public are kept low.

In the end, consumers who educate themselves on the many interrelated elements of this debate will be best equipped to decide what is right, what is wrong, and what changes are needed—even if they don't have control over the medications available to them. Educated consumers are better equipped to answer the questions presented by this debate and to propose improvements that will benefit as many people as possible. This is society's best hope for a healthy future.

GLOSSARY

aspirin   A medicine used to treat pain, fever, and swelling due to injuries, arthritis, and other inflammatory diseases.

black market   The illegal and unregulated buying and selling of substances.

clinical testing   Testing of medication on humans, which must be performed in order for a drug to gain FDA approval.

ether   A substance once used to render patients unconscious and spare them the experience of pain during surgery.

Food and Drug Administration (FDA)   The federal organization created to regulate the development and distribution of foods and medicines.

four humors The theory, popular before modern Western medicine became widespread, asserting that illness occurred when there was an imbalance in the body caused by an excess of one of the following bodily substances: yellow bile, black bile, phlegm, or blood.

insurance company An organization designed to defray certain medical costs in exchange for regular participation fees.

medications Substances intended to either aid the healing process or keep a chronic disease under control.

pharmaceutical companies Companies engaged in the research and development of new medicines and the improvement of old ones.

preclinical testing Testing of medications that is not performed on humans.

thalidomide A drug that was found to cause birth defects and was refused FDA approval in the 1960s.

FOR MORE INFORMATION

American Medical Association

http://www.ama-assn.org

The AMA is a voluntary organization for medical professionals. It publishes the *Journal of the American Medical
Association*, which is among the links on its Web site.

Bulletin of the History of Medicine

Johns Hopkins University Press

http://www.press.jhu.edu/journals/bulletin
   _of_the_history_of_medicine/toc/bhmv070.html

A good source for researching developments leading up to
the current state of medical treatment in the United States.

Centers for Disease Control and Prevention (CDC)

http://www.cdc.gov

The CDC is a part of the United States Department of

Health and Human Services. Its stated mission is to "promote health and quality of life by preventing and controlling disease, injury, and disability." The Web site presents extensive information on hundreds of diseases.

Food and Drug Administration
http://www.fda.gov
Provides in-depth information on the FDA, as well as information on many related topics and links to sites with further information.

Johns Hopkins Hospital and University
http://hopkins.med.jhu.edu
Gives the history of Johns Hopkins University and its School of Medicine and Johns Hopkins Hospital, including information on its founder, Johns Hopkins, one of the United States' most important supporters of medical research, and a listing of the inventions, discoveries, and firsts attributable to Johns Hopkins Medicine.

National Center for Complementary and Alternative Medicine
http://nccam.nih.gov
Administered by the National Institutes of Health, the NCCAM conducts research on nontraditional medical treatments and makes information available to medical professionals and the public.

NEW MEDICATIONS

National Institutes of Health
http://www.nih.gov
The NIH is another agency within the United States Department of Health and Human Services. Its focus is on research leading to better health for everyone.

National Library of Medicine
http://www.nlm.nih.gov
The world's largest medical library, featuring a collection of 5.3 million books, journals, technical reports, photos, and other items. The Web site offers access to research on health topics for both medical professionals and the public.

Pharmaceutical Research and Manufacturers of America
http://www.phrma.org
The PhRMA is a membership group for drug manufacturers. The Web site provides information on the drug approval process, the pharmaceutical industry in general, and new medications. The subsection *http://www.phrma.org/ patients/index* gives contact information on member drug companies that have programs to assist patients who cannot afford medications, along with information on eligibility and drugs included.

Thalidomide Victims Association of Canada
http://www.ogopogo.com/thalidomide

Provides information and support. Includes the TVAC's official position statement on thalidomide's return to use.

World Health Organization (WHO)
http://www.who.org
The World Health Organization works toward "the attainment by all peoples of the highest possible level of health," which it defines as "a state of complete physical, mental and social well-being and not merely the absence of disease or infirmity."

FOR FURTHER READING

Books

DeFalco, Julie C. *Treatment Delayed, Treatment Denied: Therapeutic Lag and FDA's Performance.* Washington, DC: Competitive Enterprise Institute, 1997.

Drews, Juergen, translated by David Kramer. *In Quest of Tomorrow's Medicines.* New York: Springer Verlag, 1999.

Heimann, C. F. Larry. *Acceptable Risks: Politics, Policy, and Risky Technologies.* Ann Arbor, MI: University of Michigan Press, 1998.

Higgs, Robert, ed. *Hazardous to Our Health? FDA Regulation of Health Care Products.* Oakland, CA: Independent Institute, 1995.

Mann, John. *The Elusive Magic Bullet: The Search for the Perfect Drug.* New York: Oxford University Press, 1999.

Articles

"HMO Hell." *Newsweek*, November 8, 1999, pp. 58-73.

Hunt, Terence. "Clinton Challenges Medicine Makers." *Associated Press*, October 25, 1999.

Kolata, Gina, and Kurt Eichenwald. "Stopgap Medicine: For the Uninsured, Drug Trials Are Health Care." *The New York Times*, June 22, 1999.

Pear, Robert. "Managed-Care Plans Agree to Help Pay Costs of Their Members in Clinical Trials." *The New York Times*, February 9, 1999.

Pederson, Daniel, and Eric Larson. "Too Poor to Treat." *Newsweek*, July 28, 1997.

INDEX

CREDITS

About the Author

Debbie Stanley has a bachelor's degree in journalism and a master's degree in industrial and organizational psychology.

Photo Credits

Cover photo and pp. 2, 9, 20, 37, 40, 45 © SuperStock; pp. 6, 12, 27, 30, 32, 41 © CORBIS; p. 11 © CORBIS; p. 16 © AP/Wide World Photos; p. 17 © David Forbert /SuperStock; p. 24 © Jose Luis Banus-March/FPG; p. 25 © Jeffrey Sylvester/FPG; p. 31 © Reuters/CORBIS; p. 35 by Thaddeus Harden; p. 39 by Ira Fox; p. 43 © Ralph Pleasant/FPG.

Series Design

Mike Caroleo

Layout

Laura Murawski